S's are difficult to SSaay!!

My Cancer Story

By Martin C Read

1 *This dreadful and scary disease*

This is my cancer story; it has to be "my" story because each and every one of the 300,000 plus people diagnosed with cancer every year in the UK will have a different story to tell.

My bet is, however, that for every single person who hears that dreaded sentence "You have cancer" then the first reaction, common to us all will be; FEAR.

My story from some nine months ago to today is dominated by fear, being scared, imagining all sorts of outcomes from the obvious one of death to living with some form of dreadfully curtailed lifestyle as a result of the possible treatment and potential "cure".

Fear of what has to be faced, fear of the unknown, fear of the pain to be endured, fear for those you might leave behind, fear of needles and scans and hospitals and drugs and radiology and chemotherapy and surgeons knives. A fear of job loss, a fear of income loss, a fear of not having the courage to face the future, fear of a recurrence if this cancerous tumour is not dealt with fully and fear of many other often imaginary nightmarish fears.
It gets you most when you wake up at 3.00 a.m. in the wee small hours, that is when you pray for courage, I suspect also it is when, if you are not "religious" to start with, you actually find and pray

to God; As General Storming Norman Schwarzkopf, one of the USA's most decorated soldiers once said, when asked, despite having to order the killing of many enemies and often being under serious threat of death himself, if he believed in God and if he was a religious man?, he responded by saying that "He had never met many atheists in Foxholes". I know exactly what he meant!

The other quandary and self-pitying plea I bet we all have is "Why me?" Well "Why me?" is a pretty wasted question and emotion in my view, there is no answer, no rationale. There is a temptation to review your life and question if this is some divine vengeance?

Remember: Romans 12:19–21 says,

Beloved, never avenge yourselves, but leave it to the wrath of God, for it is written, "Vengeance is mine, I will repay, says the Lord." Here we have in verse 19 the phrase, "wrath of God." "Never avenge yourselves, but leave it to the *wrath of God*, for it is written, 'Vengeance is mine, I will repay, says the Lord.'"

My view is that it is much better, no matter what previous lifetime misdemeanours made or confessions you have failed to make, is to accept that "You have it, so there is nothing you can do about it but get on and deal with it". A wise man once said that there are things in life you can do nothing about happening to you but you can always control and be in charge of your reaction to them!

For those who face the news of having cancer with aplomb and courage from the onset, you are my heroes, but I suspect there are few of you!

If this story has a purpose it is to say thank you to some very wonderful people and organisations and to provide a narrative for those who when first told the news, do what I did; desperately search for some comforting words and support as the journey to death or recovery commences. I will self-publish my story and if someone comes across it by book or on the Internet or wherever and if it provides just a modicum of comfort for them in those early days then I will feel that I "have given just a little back". I hope also that my story will offer a few imperatives for anyone who has a suspicious "lump" appear anywhere!!

The other purpose is to try and raise some donations for Cancer Research & cancer charities.

2 Finding out

So, it is nine months ago and brushing my teeth one morning I notice just a little soreness under my tongue and I guess like all big tough men, I ignore it as a small irritant, get on with the job, stop whinging, get to work, buy some mouth wash. A week later the mouthwash isn't achieving much, so let's go buy some proper mouth antiseptic, that'll do the job, well another week and of course it hasn't.

About time to actually look underneath the tongue because this" little sore" seems to be getting a life of its own and yes, there is definitely a bit of a bump there, ah well it will soon go, but of course it doesn't.

Another week and now perhaps time to tell Lynda my wonderful wife "Hey Lyn, take a look under my tongue, there's a bit of a lump which is very sore". The response is totally predictable; "I'm making an urgent appointment for you to see Doctor Sherringham". "No leave it to me I'll do it when I'm ready"; the equally predictable reply from me. Lynda never stopped asking twice daily "have you made that appointment yet?"

I have pondered long and hard over the past 9 months just why I didn't make an urgent appointment and can only conclude that I did not want to face the reality of what I think I knew - my "lump" was not natural, was not right and was probably bad news.

I then did what thousands like me do; I looked up "lump under the tongue" on the internet (some six weeks too late by now!!).

There are many sites with information, here is just one extract which after reading I knew I had to "do something" because many of the words that follow referred exactly to my symptoms (with a 50% chance of dying from it in the UK!!).

Cancer can occur in any part of the mouth, tongue, lips, throat, salivary glands, pharynx, larynx, sinus, and other sites located in the head and neck area.

How common is Mouth Cancer?

- In the UK 38,000 people are living with a diagnosis of head and neck cancer.

- Around 60,000 people in the UK will be diagnosed with mouth cancer over the next decade.

What Causes Mouth Cancer?

- Tobacco use is still considered the main cause of mouth cancer. According to the World Health Organisation, up to half of current smokers will die of a tobacco-related illness – including mouth cancer.

- Tobacco users are 6 times more likely to develop head & neck cancer.

- 75% of mouth and throat cancers occur in tobacco users.

- Alcohol is another common cause of mouth cancer. Drinking to excess can increase the risk of mouth cancer by four times.

- 3 in 4 people, who have mouth cancer, smoke and consume alcohol.

- Poor diet is linked to a third of all mouth cancer cases.

Mouth Cancer – The Facts

- Oral and pharyngeal cancer is the sixth most common malignancy reported worldwide and one with high mortality ratios among all malignancies.

- The global number of new cases was estimated at 405,318 about two-thirds of them arising in developing countries.

- Highest rates are reported in South Asian countries such as India and Sri Lanka. The Indian sub-continent accounts for one-third of the world burden.

- The incidence and mortality from oral cancer is rising in several regions of Europe, Taiwan, Japan and Australia.

- Every year in Europe, around 100,800 people are diagnosed with head and neck cancer and almost 40,000 die from the disease.

- Although there have been significant improvements in chemotherapy and surgical techniques, the disease is often particularly challenging to treat since most patients have advanced disease and secondary tumours.

- Unfortunately, 5-year survival rate has not improved (50% overall) for the last few decades, except in specialised cancer centres.

- These 'Mouth Cancers' have a higher proportion of deaths per number of cases than breast cancer, cervical cancer or skin melanoma.

- In the UK, there were 7,700 cases of mouth, throat, head and neck cancers in 2011.

- The mortality rate is just over 50%, despite treatment. Mouth cancer kills one person every 3 hours in the UK because of late detection.

- Age is another factor, with people over the age of 40 more likely to be diagnosed, though more young people are now being affected than previously.

- 25% of mouth cancer cases have no associated significant risk factors.

- Mouth cancer is twice as common in men as in women, though an increasing number of women are being diagnosed with the disease.

Mouth Cancer - The Signs and Symptoms.

In its very early stages, mouth cancers can be almost invisible making it easy to ignore. Chances of survival are improved if the cancer is detected early and rapidly treated.

It is important to have self-awareness and to perform regular, self-examinations to help in the early identification. Common symptoms include:

- A sore or ulcer in the mouth that does not heal within three weeks.

- A lump or overgrowth of tissue anywhere in the mouth.

- A white or red patch on the gums, tongue, or lining of the mouth.

- Difficulty in swallowing.

- Difficulty in chewing or moving the jaw or tongue.

- Numbness of the tongue or other area of the mouth.

- A feeling that something is caught in the throat.

- A chronic sore throat or voice change (hoarseness) that persists more than six weeks, particularly smokers over 50 years old and heavy drinkers.

- Swelling of the jaw that causes dentures to fit poorly or become uncomfortable.

- Neck swelling present for more than three weeks.

- Unexplained tooth mobility persisting for more than three weeks - see a dentist urgently.

- Persistent nasal (especially unilateral) obstruction particularly associated with mucus (clear, purulent or bloody) discharge causing difficulty breathing through nose.

- Unexplained persistent earache.

Reduce your chances of getting these cancers by:

- Not smoking or chewing tobacco, gutkha/paan.

- Limiting alcohol consumption.

- Having a healthier low meat, low fat diet, rich in vegetables and fruit with servings of bread, cereals or beans every day.

3 What to do?

Having been around pubs and the licensed trade all of my life and having been a heavy smoker up until my late 30's and a (not inconsiderable) drinker to date, I fell into some of the categories right enough!!

Now I know I have to do something and I know I have to convince Lynda that I am doing so!!

First stop "I'll go and see "Professor" Gumm. Mike Gumm is our local chemist, I call him "Professor" because he is a talented, knowledgeable, trustworthy no nonsense Chinese Australian who tells it the way it is, he is also a pal of mine. In fact, it was "Gummy" who told me that, last time I had a cancer scare, 10 years ago with a small sore on my ear that simply wouldn't heal. His words were; "well mate" (on seeing my ear for two milliseconds) "if I were you I would see Doc Sherringham by 5 o'clock tonight". That was his way of saying "look you Pratt, you've got Skin Cancer, do something about it".

I did indeed see the worthy doc that night and within 4 weeks had an operation under a local anesthetic. On reflection I now realize how flippantly I treated that little sore but as the (also) Australian consultant told me at the time "Well that's cancer mate, it won't kill you.............. well not unless it spreads that is!!"

This time it is not a small sore on the top of my ear, it is, by now a very apparent "growth" in my mouth. "Morning Professor, usual repeat prescription please" (when you get to 72 it goes with the territory I think that you end up taking 4 or 5 daily tablets of some sort or other) "give him a chair" is Gummy's usual highly amusing response.

I now ask him to take a look at this lump under my tongue and as if Déjà vu on inspection of 3 seconds he says "Well mate, if I were you I would see doc S by 5.00 p.m. tonight". He once again really meant ("look you Pratt every second you delay means a bigger problem for you cos that looks pretty nasty to me and is probably cancer!!").

Now I know I am in trouble!

Quite why I did not go home, follow Mike's advice and immediately phone the worthy doc, who I know would have seen me as an urgent case that evening, defies me to this day. I guess I simply did not want to face the reality. So I did what I guess thousands do and made an appointment in the formal way, about another 15 days lost.

"Have you made that appointment?" is Lynda's, now 3 times a day question (bordering on nagging!). "Yes, I reply", not admitting to the professor's curt advice of greater urgency; "I'm seeing Doc S in 15 days' time".

4 First steps to reality

And so the appointment day comes, the Doc takes a small torch looks under the tongue and within 3 milliseconds is making me an appointment to see a consultant at hospital, he says little to me other than "we need to get this looked at just in case it is something nasty". I knew that the speed of his pen writing out the consultancy request re affirmed my fear; "Yes, I am in trouble".

By now the lump is becoming quite sore, my speech more "throaty", my sleep is becoming more disturbed, my anxiety levels are soaring, my behaviour is becoming tetchier, my alcohol consumption is growing, my appetite is lessening, my whole well-being is going downhill fast! My imagination is running wild and my fear factor is on the highest level.

The first letter arrives, the appointment is set and in 10 days' time I have to report to the:

Oral & Maxillofacial Surgery Department at Gloucestershire Royal Hospital

I immediately look up their web site:

Welcome to our departmental website:

Oral & Maxillofacial Surgery is the medical specialty which combines surgical training with dental expertise for the treatment of diseases, injuries, tumours and deformities of the mouth, jaws and face.

Our department provides services to the population of Gloucestershire and parts of neighbouring counties.

Patients are referred to the department from both medical and dental practitioners. We also receive patient referrals from the county's two Emergency Departments if the individual has suffered facial trauma including broken jaws, cheekbones and facial lacerations.

Well it looks as though I am going to the right place, about a 45 minute journey from where we live. Ten days seems like a life time when anxiety levels are high but like all things they come to pass and they come to be.

The day comes and I set off in plenty of time, I have a sat-nav and a map. What I did not plan for was the school run, the layout of Gloucestershire Royal Hospital, the sprawling range of acreage, departments, clinics, outpatients, inpatients, around 60 departments and the car parking nightmare. I then find a car park which no-one else seems to know about, I proudly park, start walking to my destination (with little time to spare) to then find on leaving my "own" car park, a bloody great sign saying it is a dedicated car park for emergencies and any non-authorised car parked will be clamped!!

Ah, back to the car, find a helpful pedestrian and shout "hey Buddy, where is the best place to park". Predictably, in a world weary tone "In the multistory car park" is the reply. Quite how I missed a 200-foot-tall building marked "CAR PARK" is beyond me, put it down to the anxiety I guess.

Now with minutes to spare I have to find the department, this I achieve with remarkable ease and the help of some really approachable staff behind main reception (who would do justice to a 5-star hotel).

I book in and look at the waiting room clock to see that appointments are running just 10 minutes late. There are some 12 others waiting for their destinations.

Mr. Read? A smiling young nurse appears calling my name and into the consulting room we go. I am met and shake hands with the first of many (wonderful) doctors, surgeons, nurses and hospital staff I will meet over the next many months.

A preliminary chat about my symptoms and then onto the reclining chair/bed and out comes the small torch for the inspection. A second or two later comes the conclusion; "You have a tumour Mr. Read "Please call me Martin" I respond; it sadly did not change the opinion, he simply repeated; "You have a tumour Martin; we need to take a biopsy just to see what we are dealing with".

The kindly doctor then explained to me that a forthcoming conference will take a number of surgeons away for a few days which could delay the offending tumor being cut and sent for analysis. "Bear with me a second" says the worthy doc, he reappears 3 minutes later to tell me that there is a surgeon in a nearby operating theatre who can "fit me in straight away". I started to wonder if this fantastic "service" was the way the NHS works these days or whether my tumor looked so severe I would not be around to wait for any delayed analysis. Whichever way, I was taken to the theatre by my kindly Doc, introduced to Adam the surgeon, who popped me onto a bench, told me it would be like a visit to the dentist and proceeded to cut out a piece of my under- tongue. Stitches followed and we shook hands 20 minutes later with all completed!!

All done in around 35 minutes from beginning to end, fantastic, other than the fact I now know that I officially have a bloody tumour. I now also know that "I am in the system" and the administration side of the NHS will commence correspondence with me for the forthcoming many appointments.

5 *Now I know and so must others*

Back to my car with very mixed feelings, switching between; well at least I now know and can face it, too; well now I know and I might die! A very strange thing on route to my car happened; I found tears rolling down my cheeks, the first of many tears over the coming months.

The first thing to do, phone Lynda, before that however there is the huge challenge of paying the car park charges, as always I did not have enough change. So then I need to find a pay machine that takes a credit card, this is 2 floors down. I then spot a sign saying there is actually a human being in a small hut who you can talk to, give him or her a note of the realm, get your ticket stamped and leave (leave that is if you can find the exit route, or go around for an hour or two following equally lost souls).

Eventually I start on the journey home, find a lay-by just outside of town and pull in to phone Lynda.

"Hi Lyn, no easy way to say it "I have a tumour".

Lynda, a Lancashire lass, well; all in our village and our mates actually call her (fondly) a "Scouser" because she was born within the confines of that great city of Liverpool, handles the news in that brilliant way she has of being collectively; sympathetic, practical, positive, loving, whilst avoiding the obvious rollicking of saying "I'd told you to go earlier".

We talked for a few minutes more and she would be waiting for me to give me a cuddle and plan our fight back from here on in. She of course did leave me with the thought "It might well be non-malignant/benign, let's not over worry before we know what we are dealing with". What a gal.

I call into my beloved sister Josephine to tell her the news and that is not such an easy conversation, I struggled more than she but I'm afraid a few more tears flowed from me.

We also have to inform our beautiful daughter Georgina what is happening. Georgie had texted Lynda during the day asking "do I need to prepare myself for when I get home?" (She is 19 going on 45 in wisdom). "No honey, dad will tell you all, but don't worry".

I did see G when she arrived home from school. "G, I have a tumour which could be cancerous, so if it is, we will just have to battle through it". She took the news just like the trooper she is. No tears from G, only me. Lynda has since told me of Georgina's tears when she went to bed that night. I am so pleased that I did not see them.

6 Doctors, consultants, nurses, heroes

The first letter arrived a day or two later confirming an appointment with a Mr. Mark Singh BDS (Lon)
MFDS RCS (Eng) MBBS (UWI) MRCS (Eng) FRCS (OMFS). I look him up on Google and I am immediately impressed;

Consultant in Oral and Maxillofacial Surgery, Areas of expertise; Head and Neck Surgery Oral & Maxillofacial Surgery Oncology Salivary glands, Skin malignancy.

This sounds like the guy for me!!

I'm coming with you says Lynda, I know you, you will only listen to the good bits and ignore what you are being told to do, I give in and we await the fateful day.

We meet Mr Singh for the first time and we shake hands. Now; I have been around a long time in life and business and I instinctively know a hand shake accompanied with profound eye contact that tells me I am dealing with a man of substance, character and trust. For me; Intelligence and charisma flowed out of this man after just 2 minutes of contact.

Lynda and I sat opposite him, with a nurse in the background of the consulting room.

"We have the results of your biopsy Mr Read" (please call me Martin) once again this personal acquaintance effort did not change the news. Your tumour is cancerous, so you have cancer".

A more technical description followed which I didn't really take in too closely! "How do you react to that diagnosis Martin?" "Well I'm scared, worried and frankly bloody disappointed I'd rather hoped you would say that it had proven to be benign! I do however trust you guys implicitly and so I put myself entirely in your hands".

"That's a good attitude Martin, now let me explain what we can do for you, but first let me tell you that this is not an automatic death sentence, we see and treat many people each year with your condition and many of our patients make a full recovery and go on to lead normal lives", I noticed that he said "many" rather than "all".

Then, out came a bit of A4 paper and I immediately thought, this Mr Singh is a man after my own heart, keep it simple, communicate in a way people can understand, avoid being clever using long medical words, tell it the way it is, he also wanted me to know that I would not be treated as a "patient" but more as a customer!! Gee whiz the NHS are fabulous!

Mr Singh proceeded in a very professional but certainly objective way to explain, by scribing on the piece of paper in front of him; "So here we have your tongue, with the tumour underneath, we do not know at this stage how far the cancer has spread, so what we will do is send you for an X ray, find out if it has spread and see if it's gone elsewhere and then decide where to cut".

"If it is just a cut around the area we think it's in, then, we will over-cut so we have a better likelihood of getting it all, then we will cut out a piece of your arm, with veins and artery, which we will stitch into the missing part of the tongue we have cut out, this will also be over-sized because it shrinks over a period of 6 months or so. We will then cut a line across your throat, take out all of your lymph nodes and then microscopically plumb in the veins and artery so that the arm part gets blood and oh yes we might have to break your Jaw to get at it all and of course we will cut out a piece of your tummy to replace the piece out of your arm".

I was tempted to say "if you ever get any good news don't hesitate to phone!"

"Any questions Martin?"

I looked at Lynda who gave a pretty Scouse comment, something like" Well that should get the little bugger".

My questions and comments were a little more practical I think "Thanks for the detail Mr Singh but tell me for my first question; there is always a DO NOTHING option, so tell me, if I decide on that, what IS LIKELY TO HAPPEN?"

"You are of course correct Martin, "do nothing" could be your choice, it is your body and life after all, so if you choose that route here is what we know; Tumours of the nature that you have, continue to grow, they are unstoppable, so it will over a period of an undetermined time span, become a walnut, then a golf ball, then an orange. It will be at some stage probably between golf ball and orange that you are likely to choke to death".

That cheered me up no end!

Question two; "will I be able to talk afterwards?"(I was terrified that they might cut out my voice box).

26

"Well" said Mr Singh, "you will have difficulty in speaking for a month or two, bit like this"; he then gave a sort of lousy ventriloquist's version of a dummy under water, "but don't worry with some speech therapy and 6 months' practice; most of my patients (customers) regain total oratory skills as before". Again I would have preferred ALL rather than MOST.

"One more question Mr Singh; this x-ray you mention; I am not going to have to go into one of those "tubes" am I?" I need to tell you that I am somewhat claustrophobic (ever since being trapped whilst pot-holing some years ago on a ridiculous corporate team building exercise, which destroyed team spirit for ever more and ensured that one of my fellow "trapped" colleagues had to endure counselling for many months).

"Don't worry" says he, "I will let them know and we will ask for the "more open one" for you".

"Where's the bit of paper to sign?"

He produced a piece of A4 with details of:

The planned procedure, assessment of the health professional, the serious or recurring risks and lots of other "due diligence" items and then a place for my signature agreeing to the procedure.

I signed...........................

Fate sealed!!!

"Oh, just before we leave" Mr Singh, "would there be a previous patient of yours who has gone through what I have to go through and might be prepared to talk to me to give their perspective on the matter". "Oh yes absolutely" says he and gives me the e-mail address of a person called Lea.

7 *And so it starts*

Next letter arrives for the first x-ray appointment, off to Cheltenham this time, fearing just how "open" this machine would be.

As it turned out, it really was "open(ish)" so no problem, job done in 20 minutes.

Next letter arrives a few days later with an appointment to see Mr Singh again.

Lynda and I turn up on the due day and time, see Mr Singh along this time with his colleague Mr Godden. "First piece of good news Martin is that the x-ray has established that the cancer has not spread and is localised to the mouth/throat area". We sigh with relief.

"So let's get you on the table and have a look at how we can go about things".

I lie down and the two experts who will save my life start discussing the mechanics of the procedure.

"Perhaps break it here?" I hear, "Hang on boys, break what say I?" "Your Jaw Martin", bloody Hell think I.

"Or perhaps just remove the teeth, we could then go in that way".

Bloody Hell say I?"

How many boys?"

"I would say 6 or 7!!

It was at that stage I was rather hoping that any of those to be removed would not be the ones I have paid £6k to have implanted some 5 years ago.

Mr S and Mr G continued to debate various aspects of the forthcoming operation and I am sure I detected some sense of quiet excitement in their voices at what was going to be a 12 hour procedure, testing every one of their skills or more and their past 20 odd years of qualifications. For me there was little sense of shared excitement!

Consultation over, the next piece of news was that a further more detailed x-ray of the localised area was needed prior to the operation date which was agreed to be in just two weeks' time. Mr S did explain that this x-ray would be a "tube" job but he would arrange for a specialist place to go where they have the latest and "most open under the circumstances equipment."

So I now had two weeks before going into hospital to test my theory that "I trust you guys implicitly!" Prior to that of course I had the ordeal of the next more enclosed x-ray to face.

8 Start planning & telling

We returned home, now knowing that in two weeks' time my life would change and so the new challenge arises. Who do we tell? What do we tell them? Also; what do we do about the business we run?

Firstly, we have to tell Georgina which proved to be very difficult for me and I think privately for G. Lynda told me that despite her courage in front of me during our conversation, she later "broke her heart" when in her room that night. It was one of my original fears of hurting other people especially those closest to me. Once again I am so pleased that I did not witness those tears.

Without boring you dear reader about our business which is dedicated to the Licensed trade (more alcohol involved I'm afraid), we decided that Lynda (who is part of the business anyway) would take on my role as MD, come onto the board of our limited company and I would take a "back seat" for the next 6 months at least (she would say it hasn't worked out that way!!). This involved communicating with a fellow director and staff of our company, telling them the truthful reason, all were incredibly supportive and we received some of the most touching letters and messages, more tears fell I am afraid.

Stage three in the "telling" process is of course "family and friends". (I have no doubt that some of the other 300,000 sufferers take a different course and decide to tell no one, it is a very personal choice and I think there is no right or wrong way of dealing with it).

Our family and friends are told and once again you realise just how blessed you are to have such wonderful support. Different people handle this sort of news in different ways, my mates decided a load of pub visits and dinner parties squeezed in to two weeks would bolster me up a bit for the battle ahead, remarkable how you can gain about half a stone in two weeks! Love and affection in abundance from true friends and family helped me prepare for the battle. I learned that big tough rugby lads can also cuddle you and show a wet eye themselves and that girlfriends can kiss you in a way that reminds you of how motherly instincts are primeval in their warmth.

The list is too long to record here, but each of those wonderful, friends, family members, neighbours and work mates know who they are and know that they have my eternal love and thanks for their kindness towards me and also their great support for Lynda.

The dreaded letter arrives for the next x-ray, this time I am to attend the (wonderful) Cobalt Centre in Cheltenham; I immediately view their web site:

Founded in 1964, Cobalt is an independent medical charity helping people affected by cancer, dementia and other life-limiting conditions. Each year we provide diagnostic imaging for over 24,000 patients at Cobalt Imaging Centre in Cheltenham and with our mobile MRI (Magnetic Resonance Imaging) scanners that travel throughout the Three Counties (Gloucestershire, Herefordshire, Worcestershire) and beyond.
We offer free training and education courses on a local, national and international basis

for doctors and healthcare professionals,
ensuring our experience and research work is
widely shared. We also visit local schools,
companies and organisations delivering free
cancer prevention and health education
talks.

Donations we receive help fund scanning and
diagnosis, research, prevention, specialised
nursing posts and cancer facilities for local
people. For every £1 of our total diagnostic
and voluntary income we spend 88p on our
charitable work.

We have a proud history of fundraising
achievements. We have been a major NHS
partner in establishing the Oncology Centre
at Cheltenham General Hospital and other
health care facilities, such as the £5.1 million,
all digital, Thirlestaine Breast Centre at
Cobalt House. Check out our history page
which has details of some of the significant
projects we have helped with over the years.
We are dedicated to providing patients and
other hospitals with better access to
diagnostic services such as MRI, PET/CT,

CT, X-ray and Ultrasound. By continuing to improve efficiency, we help to drive down prices too. Our unique diagnostic centre offers MRI scanning, at a variety of magnetic strengths (measured in Teslas), on different magnets and fields. We have the UK's first high field open MRI, a 3.0 Tesla MRI on site at the Imaging Centre and we also have a fleet of six mobile MRIs including several 1.5 Tesla MRI and Europe's first 3.0 Tesla mobile MRI. Our scanners receive software and hardware upgrades regularly to incorporate advancements in technology. We have recently invested in a brand new, state of the art PET/CT Scanner, which has been especially designed to improve patient comfort, shorten scanning times and provide exceptional image quality.

We undertake and fund research projects that bring tangible benefits to patients affected by cancer and other life-limiting conditions, and we work closely with our NHS colleagues to bring about improvements to the treatment of these illnesses. Cobalt's Cancer Prevention Service helps to educate the public by providing clear accurate messages to help people make informed personal lifestyle choices.

We support the NHS breast cancer screening programme with specialist scans for young and 'at risk' patients, for whom mammography is not appropriate.

■ ■

I particularly liked this sentence;

We have recently invested in a brand new, state of the art PET/CT Scanner, which has been especially designed to both, improve patient comfort, shorten scanning times and provide exceptional image quality.

9 Support

At around this time and with about 10 days to go before entering hospital I am now really scared, so I seek whatever solace I can and search for support groups or the like. I come across the (wonderful) charity known as Maggie's; this is a small extract from their website:

People with cancer need places like these

Every year, over 300,000 people are diagnosed with cancer in the UK, facing tough questions, exhausting treatment and difficult emotions. These challenges affect not only those with cancer, but their family and friends, too.

Maggie's is there for anyone and everyone affected by cancer, offering a programme of support that has been shown to strengthen physical and emotional wellbeing.

Built alongside the hospital, our Centres are uplifting places with professional staff on hand to offer the support people need: practical advice about benefits and eating well; emotional support from qualified experts; a friendly place to meet other people; a calming space simply to sit quietly with a cup of tea.

The National Cancer Survivorship Initiative Report by the Department of Health in 2013 highlights our unique approach to cancer care as example of best practice. Since 2000 our work has also been commended by the NHS Cancer Plan, NICE and the Cancer Reform Strategy.

Last year Maggie's received 125,000 visits and supported over 25,000 people newly affected by cancer; among our visitors 99% found the support we offer helpful.

I visit Maggie's and find the kindest most helpful people in the world, I meet also fellow sufferers, enjoy a cup of tea and a piece of cake and leave the centre knowing there is a safe place to return to whenever I feel the need to find solace.

I also send an email (MR Singh's referral) to "Lea", we miss each other a couple of times but eventually speak by telephone. I hear this lady who has the most infectious laughter in her voice, diction that would bless a Shakespearean actress, enthusiasm that would inspire an Army going into battle and then by sheer coincidence a shared knowledge and friendship with a pub landlord!

During our conversation which has drifted from cancer to commerce, we also discover that we operate in a similar business sector and that perhaps when my plight is redeemed we should meet to see if we can do business together!

I reflect on the call and on subsequent emails, that Mr Singh was right "many of my patients recover completely!" and that how small the world really is. I am bolstered by my contact with Lea.

10 Courage mon brave

My next x-ray appointment day arrives and I turn up, wait no more than 15 minutes and in I go to the x-ray room, very kind attendees show me "the machine "and it looked mightily "closed" to me! They explain the procedure; I will go in head first, full length, stay in for around 50 minutes, stay completely still, suffer extremely loud noises but I am assured by them; "it can't hurt you".

"I'm claustrophobic I pathetically cry out".

Don't worry Mr Read (I didn't offer the option of "Martin") "you can hold a panic button and any time you want to stop, just press it and we will come in to release you".

Bloody Hell I thought?!

I was laid out, ear plugs in, foam pressed against my temples, a kind of clamp pressed to the foam, a kind of hoop lowered onto my skull, a button pressed and in I went!!

The machine started, the (unbelievable) noise commenced and my heart rate went to stratospheric levels, strangely enough whilst the noise was going on I felt (reasonably) ok. I knew something was going on and so I knew it was part of my treatment and was designed to help me. It was in the intervals that the noise stopped (presumably to line up more x-ray plates) that "panic in the silence" gave me the opportunity to think too much and to realise that I could not move or escape.

The definition for claustrophobia is; an abnormal fear of enclosed places.

I agree with that!

Pathetically after about 10 minutes I press the panic button and out I come with the nurses having rushed into the room.

"I'm sorry Guys, I don't think I can do this, I need some form of relaxant or knock out drug".

Don't worry Mr Read, quite a number of our patients have a challenge with this, we can arrange another date for you and prior to the date help you with a little anxiety potion".

"That's great say I, when can the date be?

Around three to four weeks' time".

"Oh dear say I, I am due in hospital for my operation in around 6 days", "well that gives us two choices, go back in and try again or delay your operation".

Not much of a choice really, I go back in, I sing in my head: "My way" along with "Always look on the bright side of life" and "You'll never walk alone". Somehow the next 40 minutes pass and I shall be eternally grateful to Frank Sinatra, The life of Brian and Gerry and the Pacemakers!!

The task finished and I think I can honestly say I have never been more relieved when the button was pressed to allow my escape (well only slightly less so than when we escaped from that pot hole 25 years ago!!).

On the way out of the x-ray room, I passed the next "victim" waiting with what I thought was a very anxious look on her face "don't worry" said I; "it's a piece of cake!!"

I was also able that night in the local pub to tell my mates how brave I had been (I didn't mention the premature pressing of the panic button!).

11 In I Go

Days come and days go and eventually the day of admission to the Gloucestershire Royal Hospital arrives, we have an arrival time booked of 7.00am!

We leave home with Lynda driving at 6.05, leaving our beloved daughter Georgina asleep as I have said my goodbyes to her the night before. I privately prayed that it would not be the last time I saw her.

We are there before the staff arrive (Lynda has no problem finding car parking) and we are first in the queue to enter the pre-op reception office. A kindly nurse appears and in we go to a private screen area. There is much documentation to complete, kit to be taken off, operating gown to be put on, nervous glances twixt Lynda and me. You are first on Martin so any minute now we will get you onto a bed (still not too late, shall I do a runner?) no chance with Lynda holding my day clothes.

Ten minutes go by and a new nurse appears to wheel me into the operating theatre, now I am resigned to my fate, trust these people is all I can think. I kiss Lynda goodbye and I'm now wheeled in to meet the Anaesthetist and his team.

"Hi Mr Read, we are here to look after you, are you allergic to anything?" Yes, say I; Oysters! "You will be safe from them here" says he!

I feel one of the team doing something with my right arm and I wake up two and half days later!!

12 *I'm still alive*

"I'm still awake, I'm still awake", these are the first words I utter (well utter is an exaggeration, more these are the first words I think I mumbled). I had this strange sensation that I was still with the anaesthetic team and they were about to operate with me still wide awake! (I had read somewhere about twenty years ago that a lady had been anesthetised but had stayed awake throughout the entire procedure of her operation but had not been able to communicate that to the surgeon, bloody scary!)

"Yes you are awake Martin and it's all over, you have had your operation" said my specialist nurse in the critical care unit. I couldn't believe it!! (I also could not believe it later when Lynda told me that following my eleven-hour operation (shorter than expected) and being placed into the unit, I was wheeled back into the operating theatre on the following day because my blood pressure had dropped to a dangerously low level, the surgeons once again performed their magic and somehow I was put into an even deeper sleep to see my blood pressure get back to an acceptable level. Lynda had apparently been telephoned from the actual operating theatre and was no doubt very worried about my chances of survival.

So; on finally re-awakening after two visits to the surgeons I saw the best sight in the world; Lynda and what do you know her sister Carolyn who lives in Brussels. "Hi Mart" says Cal, "I hope you are OK with me being here, I just had to come over to support "our Lyn" whilst you are in hospital". I could not have been more pleased.

The next day or two passed and if I am honest I have very little recollection of what happened. I do recall struggling to breath, which I thought was a pretty essential part I had to play in my survival. My dedicated nurse in critical care was just that; dedicated and eventually, I think on day three (maybe four) I was moved to a private room in ward 2B.

13 Start the recovery, get a summary of events!

Mr Singh had always told me that recuperation and hospital stay would be around fourteen days and so I steeled myself to handle my self-pity (which I am pretty good at; self-pity that is; not handling it) for that sort of duration.

Adam, one of the medical team called in on me and explained that I was not to move my head to the right for some 3 or 4 days and that, it was now down to me to recover, "we have done what we had to do Martin and now the next 10 days or so will be critical to your recovery, boredom and the physiological side of things is what you now have to deal with. Plenty of TV, reading and whatever else you can do to fill the time is essential".

Lynda and Cal were with me in that private room along with my sister and gave me every piece of encouragement, I just whinged and cried a lot! (I am told that emotion often follows a major operation (especially eleven hours of it!!).

I guess we are at day 5 by now and Lynda tells me that Georgina is due later to see me. Please don't let her see me like this I plead. I knew I looked like a car crash victim; swollen head twice the normal size, blood leaking around mouth and throat, dark shadows under my eyes, stubble of four days' growth, weeping frequently, a bit smelly, full of self-pity, blood spots on my pyjama top.

"Believe me says Lynda, "You look a bloody site better than the first time she saw you". I was amazed, "When was that" say I "On day one after your operation, we three came in and compared to that time you look like Brad Pitt". I simply could not believe that Georgie had handled such a traumatic scene, it was then I realised what love and character can handle.

"You have to be strong for her visit" says Cal and incredibly I was (I think). It was only when the time came for them all to leave I reverted to my pathetic pathos.

The days passed so slowly, the TV was my friend, my mobile phone my contact with the outside world (text not calls!!) my I Pad my pastime! The (wonderful) nurses my heroes, my Oxygen mask my means of surviving and my books my challenge to concentrate upon. Many of my pals asked to visit, but Lynda being Lynda knew I was not up to it and so acted as my Gatekeeper, the visits, however, from family (who would accept my miserableness, moaning, inability to speak coherently and my demands and self-pity): Lynda, Cal, Georgina, my sister, Bro in law, Alan and Paulene (who had come up to stay with Lynda from Burnham on Sea in the latter two days) were my anticipation and excitement.

Those visits meant so much and never seemed to last long enough, I fell in to a sadness whenever they left and could only wish for time to speed up for their return, I also longed to see my buddies but that had to wait until my release.

I simply resolved myself to one task; just take the next breath. This on occasions was easier said than done and in honesty I can say that there were perhaps three or four occasions when I panicked that the next breath would not come and that I might die! There were also perhaps a few occasions that I wished it would not do so (the next breath that is), but the human spirit and survival instinct is much stronger than human flesh!!

14 More drama

"I am sorry Martin but we are going to have to move you to a public ward".

I didn't receive the news with any great enthusiasm, quite why not I am not sure about, perhaps I thought I was special in some way, I soon learned that I was not.

I arrived in the public ward to find just a four bed room, I gave the thumbs up sign to the guy opposite me and he returned the gesture, it was late and I tried (unsuccessfully) to sleep. In fact, sleeping became a major difficulty over the following four or five days, primarily due to the after effects of the anaesthetic, mucus, sore throat, phlegm, coughing, night time activity in the ward, listening to your fellow roommates trying to stay alive and constant re-awakening by the nurses to give you something to help you sleep!!

The early morning ward visit of the surgery team led by Mr Godden (Mr Singh had a few days off but was kept updated by screen shots taken of my healing), about six strong, meant more probing and inspection of my new tongue, throat area, scars, nose feeding tube and the regular question; "how are you feeling?" (My reply ranged from "lousy" to unrepeatable Anglo Saxon but I like to think that I was always gracious and appreciative!). Then on a visit on about day six came the shattering news; "Martin, we are going to have to take you back into the operating theatre". "Oh no" say I; "why?"

"Well", says Mr Godden, "the few remaining teeth you have are starting, involuntarily, to chew on the skin graft on your tongue and it looks like a small infection is happening we will need to trim the skin area so that it stops".

I dread the thought of another operation and dread the thought that it will keep me from going home even longer.

"There is an option to have the procedure carried out by way of a local anaesthetic", says Mr Godden, "what are the implications of that?" Say I.

"Well it will be a bit like going to the dentist and of course because you will be awake throughout, it will be less traumatic than general anaesthetic and will not "put you back as much" in terms of your recovery or release date".

"That's the one for me" say I (bravely but stupidly?).

I am not sure which dentist the surgeons have received treatment from over the years but whichever one it is he or she will struggle to make a living or have many repeat customers!

In I go. Local anaesthetic applied, then the "trimming starts", pulling, pushing, widening of the mouth, getting to the offending skin, more pushing, more pulling, more stretching and with trimming of course also comes more stitching and then (worst) of all comes the re-placement of the nose tube that feeds me.

Now; the pushing down of a thin tube into the tummy is known as:

> Nasogastric (NG) intubation - a procedure during which a thin, plastic tube is inserted through the nostril, down the esophagus, and into the stomach. Once an NG tube is in place, healthcare providers can deliver food and medicine directly to the stomach or remove substances from it. Nasogastric (NG) intubation is most often used to deliver food and medicine to a patient when they are unable to eat or swallow.

All sounds good and simple? Well it aint!!

Following the trimming exercise and still in the operating theatre and ten minutes after trying unsuccessfully to push down the tube, with me retching, choking and coughing, my surgeon decides "He's had enough for now, we will do it later".

Later turns out to be around midnight, more retching, choking and coughing accompanies the attempt which eventually goes in! This has to be followed by a visit to the x-ray department to ensure it is in the right place (stomach not lungs).

I wait for the porter to take me to the x-ray department (a long wait). I ask the nurse tetchily "how much longer do I have to wait" (it is now about 3.00am). The reply humbles me somewhat "there has been a serious crash on the M5 and I'm afraid finding out if your tube is in the right place is rather low down on the priority list" I accept the wait.

Eventually I have the x-ray, the result comes an hour or so later; "It's in the wrong place". Out it comes and once more I "suffer" the next (dreaded) attempt to get it down, this time it does go down a little easier because the next person to try gives me a tip to try and swallow retained water in the mouth as the push to go pass the esophagus happens. Back to the x-ray department and the result now shows Hurray "it's in the right place"!!

Now at last they can fix me up with some sustenance going into my tummy. It starts feeding me and unbelievably after just one feeding bag of whatever is in such a bag, a bit of a sneeze saw the whole bloody tube fly out of my nose like a jet plane!!

We will have to put it back in says the Doc.

I'm pretty sure that up until now, I have been a reasonably good patient, now however I get a bit seriously tetchy! "I'm not, repeat not, going through that again, categorically". "Well" says the worthy Doc, "the only way we can avoid that and feed you is by you eating and swallowing yourself" (which up until then I had really struggled with). I am informed in no uncertain manner that I must prove that I can drink two litres of water a day and eat three meals! No problem says I!!

Now a confession; I did eat and I did drink, but I also found a way of tipping half of the required minimum into various receptacles around the ward and by recruiting the help of my next door bed neighbour to tip some of my ration into his receptacles (you can create good mates in times of difficulty). I did feel a scintilla of guilt each time a nurse (who had to record my consumption) praised my intake!

15 Upwards and onwards

There comes a time of course when the bed you have occupied for your first few days becomes the nurses' great challenge to get you out of!

"Time you got out of bed and started walking around a bit Martin" and so I gingerly (very) swing a leg out and grab hold of my feeding tube stand which will become my support for those early steps. Well actually you ask the kindly nurse to support you! But then after six or seven steps I let go of the nurses' steadying hand and gee whiz, I am walking unaided, well plus my "on wheels" support stand. Off I go on an adventure into the corridor and up and down that passageway looking in on other patients and intimating hello to anyone capable of seeing or answering. I feel like a North Pole trekker but soon after two trips up and down the corridor of about 50 meters in total, I retire back to bed pretty exhausted.

This new found independence allows me to visit the bathroom for a wash and shave; the latter I abandoned after two pulls on my razor, in favour of growing a beard, somewhat to make life easier, somewhat to hide my scars but mostly to stop the pain those first two pulls inflicted!

The new found independent bathroom trip is replaced by another kindly nurse who offers me a personal "wash down" warts and all, which I accepted with alacrity, this proved to be just a one-off offer and service.... shame.

It occurred to me that my sister might have a walking stick in a cupboard somewhere and a text message to her saw the article delivered on her next visit. I observed the stick with familiarity as it was the very walking stick my dear old recently departed Mum had used during her time towards the end of her long life in a nursing home. So here I was using the family walking stick to aid my now frequent trips up and down the corridor and seeing that my mum was ninety-six when she passed on, I could not help but reflect that getting older is no fun, let alone getting older with cancer as your curse! The walking stick did provide me with the opportunity to turn it into a pretend Banjo and when passing nurses in the corridor I would strum away on it to their (I hope) amusement but also perhaps to their concern that I should be moved to a more suitable ward for disturbed patients!

It did however persuade me that I might no longer be able to speak that well, my sense of humour had not been removed with my tongue!

16 The heroes

It did occur to me that those fabulous nurses, in addition to keeping patients alive with injections, feeding, pain killers, changing beds, emptying pee bottles, dealing with emergencies, chasing to answer panic buttons, and a thousand other tasks, usually over a twelve-hour shift, seemed to spend most of their time, when not saving lives; filling in bloody forms! The thickness of my Folder kept at the end of my bed would have done justice to a re write of War and Peace!

"Well done Martin" would be the praise as the chart was updated with my excellent appetite and liquid intake. I merely nodded that I was doing my best! I did reach the conclusion, however, that if a body gets hungry enough and thirsty enough, then natural survival instincts will find a way for food and water to be consumed!

Whilst I have previously mentioned that moving to a public ward from a private ward, somewhat disappointed me, the experience of sharing with three other "sufferers" proved; that no matter how much or little money you have, no matter what status you have achieved in life, no matter what big house or little house you live in, suffering from cancer will level you out to what we all are: human beings with an illness that can (and for one fellow sufferer I am sure soon did) kill you. There is no "point scoring" when you are at risk of death, there is a strange almost unspoken bond that happens immediately you see fellow sufferers (most suffering much more than me!).

I had two long term (5 day) fellow patients in my ward and three short term guys who were "in and out" in short shift.

My two fellow "lifers "(5 days) and I soon developed a sort of Morse code or Semaphore system, thumbs up; good day, thumbs down; bad day, arms flapping; when you going home?" and so on. Both of my new mates sadly had it much worse than me and had lost their voice boxes and so would probably never speak again. I just could not be imaging the horror of such a predicament. We all had pens and writing pads (my speech was pretty limited for most of this time) and we spent many hours dropping each other a note on a wide range of subjects. It is amazing how much you can find out about a person over such a small period of time and with such limited means of communication. I do not know of their fate, because, I left them in their beds on my departure, we shook hands and wished each other well with our code, I trust they have found some way of coping.

There was one moment of high drama in the ward, when "Harry" (I have changed his real name because he was a co-conspirator in my food disposal deceit) was due to be discharged but had to have a catheter removed prior to his release. The doctor arrived, drew the curtain around Harry's bed and was chatting to him quite normally, when all of a sudden the doctor's voice rose alarmingly "Can you hear me Harry, Harry can you hear me, nurse press the bell I need help here". The bell rang and from somewhere appeared at least three nurses and two further doctors. I heard "We are losing him, we are losing him", this along with other commands to do things and then suddenly Harry kind of coughed or spluttered and said "yes I can hear you" I think they saved his life in those ten minutes!

I saw Harry later on that evening and there was no way he was going home!!

17 Longing to go home

Visits from Lynda, Georgina, my sister Josephine and B in Law Lee continued (Cal had returned to Brussels having supported Lynda for a wonderful week) and a quick one-off visit from Alan and Paulene (who I have known for over 40 years) were great occasions throughout my stay. In the early days I had difficulty in speaking for long periods and so my note book and pen would be furiously used. I have retained the note book and have studied the cryptic notes which seem to contain a tremendous number of Anglo Saxon expletives and I am now, on re-reading the script, unable to understand much of what I was asking for, commenting on or trying to describe. I can only imagine that my visitors somehow worked out what I was trying to say!

On day ten, I was visited as usual by the surgical team led by Mr. Godden, inspection of my mouth, my scarred arm, my tummy scar and speech took place and a demonstration of my, by now, quite (relatively) sophisticated method of swallowing and eating was demanded. "That's fine"

said the top man "You can go home tomorrow".
Very sweet words I assure you!

I was ready and dressed to depart by 9.30 on day eleven, this proved to be rather optimistic as there are many procedures and administration to go through before any patient (customer) is discharged. Three p.m. however eventually arrives and the most wonderful sight of Lynda coming to" rescue me" appears. I say my goodbyes to my ward mates and those fabulous doctors and nurses who have cared for me.

18 Home

On arrival home, Lynda shows me into my "recuperation room". We are lucky enough to have at home a Garden Room which Lynda has fixed up with a bed, internet, laptop, phone charger, bedside table that extends over the bed, tissues, tablets, medicine, Get Well Cards, books, golf magazines, box sets, new pajamas, dressing gown, slippers, extra pillows, high tog duvet and a Welcome Home sticker!

Home after just eleven days from my first 7.00 a.m. arrival at hospital, about nine months' from that first little sore under my tongue; I sleep an afternoon sleep for three hours; wonderful!

When I awaken, I have to remind myself; you have had cancer, you might still have some remnants, you might need radiotherapy or chemotherapy, the battle isn't over, you have a piece of your arm stitched into your mouth, you cannot speak properly, you no longer have a functioning tongue, you have some pain and soreness, it is not over yet!! There are many more hospital appointments to come. BUT Hey "I'm alive!!!"

19 Great news and a future

On my 72nd birthday I have my first review session with Mr. Singh and if you want the best birthday present you have ever had, go see Mr. Singh and be told (I paraphrase) "We got it all, you no longer have cancer" I want to hug him!

So the long journey of healing has begun, more hospital visits ahead, no doubt more x-rays to check wellbeing, more trimming of the tongue ahead, more attempts to speak coherently , more dressings for the injured arm (stitches have been removed by my wonderful specialist nurse) more psychological battles to adapt to knowing "I am not the man I was" more teeth to be replaced, more bruising to subside, more patience to accept I am relatively inactive, more time to elapse before I can play golf again, more practice to get back to enjoying a pint of bitter, more displeasure at eating and tasting properly, more effort to keep warm , more worry about catching a cold, more weight to try and regain (or stop losing). More practice at being kind to those caring for me , more time ahead to live with this "foreign body in my mouth" the fear has, however, been replaced with HOPE and I have overcome any embarrassment about my gummy noteeth appearance when I meet friends. Being alive with no teeth, slurred speech a new fluffy beard to hide my scars is much better than the alternative!

Many cards and emails flood my way and so I composed a simple script when asked "what happened? Here it is...............

I am home after not the best few weeks of my life but at least still above ground.
I try to avoid "war stories" about my operation but in essence.........
To save my life; they took out most of my tongue and throat (now in a waste bin) cut out part of my arm with veins and artery attached, sowed that lot . into my mouth, avoided breaking my jaw to get at the cancer but took out my teeth (including the ones I recently paid £6k for) so it was easier for them to get to the cancer, cut out part of my belly to replace the piece out of the arm, put a 10 inch scar across my throat to remove all lymph nodes, took me back to the operating theatre the following day because my blood pressure dropped to dangerously low level, and then operated a third time to cut down the piece of arm in my mouth because it was too big and I couldn't breathe (which I found to be an essential factor in surviving).

The first thing they then ask you after you have been "out" for 3 days is "How are you feeling". I will avoid repeating my response!

Good news at the moment is that "they got it all" and so I have the all clear until the next review in a months' time.

I can just about make myself understood with what feels like an orange glued into my gob

But Speech Therapy follows over the next few weeks; however, it might be a while however before my next pubic speaking engagement! They say it could have been caused by too much Alcohol and Smoking over the years (unlikely in my view).

20 The plan

So the plan is "be patient, sleep a lot, try to regain 2 stone weight loss, take 6 months to heal, try to learn to talk again, reduce alcohol intake, don't take up smoking again, take loads of pills, be kind to those looking after you, all of which leaves me bored out of my brains!! But Lynda is doing a great job as MD (I will probably become "Chairman").

21 They are fabulous!

Just one serious note "The NHS are the Dogs Bollocks" Fabulous, Sensational and Bloody Marvellous.

So dear reader nine months of my life have gone by, perhaps a year ahead to get back to some normality. I hope my little story has given an insight into an experience I trust none of you will have to endure. I hope also that anyone reading this tome will not now delay one second if they find a "lump" anywhere!

22 Getting used to a new me

My first "public outing" minus teeth and with my orange in my mouth was to the local church carol service and what do you know the first carol was "Whilst Shepherds watch their Sheep at night". My second trip out was a lunch; when I ordered "Soup please", only for the waiter to say "pardon Sir?" I now know so much more than I knew before; Firstly, I know that S's are difficult to say!!

I know that I have been one of the lucky ones. I know others will not survive the way I have. I know if any sign of "a lump" is dealt with more quickly, your chances of recovery will be enhanced.
I know the NHS is wonderful. I know my family, friends and neighbours are fabulous, I know my wife and daughter are more than fabulous, I know the human spirit is unconquerable, I know all men are equal. I do not know but I now suspect that there is a God. I know my extended family are tremendous. I know others suffered and are suffering more than me. I know my life has changed. I know there is support out there. I know Mr Godden, Mr Singh and their team are from

heaven. I know I need to find a way to say thank you properly to so many people. I know courage can be found if the fright is great enough. I know that there is nothing to fear but fear itself. I know nurses aren't paid enough. I know the spirit is stronger than flesh. I know the NHS is and should be the envy of the world! I know that this vicious, hateful disease must be conquered; I know that this can only be achieved by way of research. I know research costs money and so whatever "profit" there is after production cost of this book, such profit will be donated to Cancer Research & cancer charities.

But most of all I know that being alive is great!

Post Script

Since my writing of this little tome, my daughter, unbeknown to me, has Blogged on her perspective of "her Dad having cancer". I read it ten minutes ago and I am still crying as I read her words.

Here is G's story........

His story, through my eyes.

Georgina Forsyth-Read

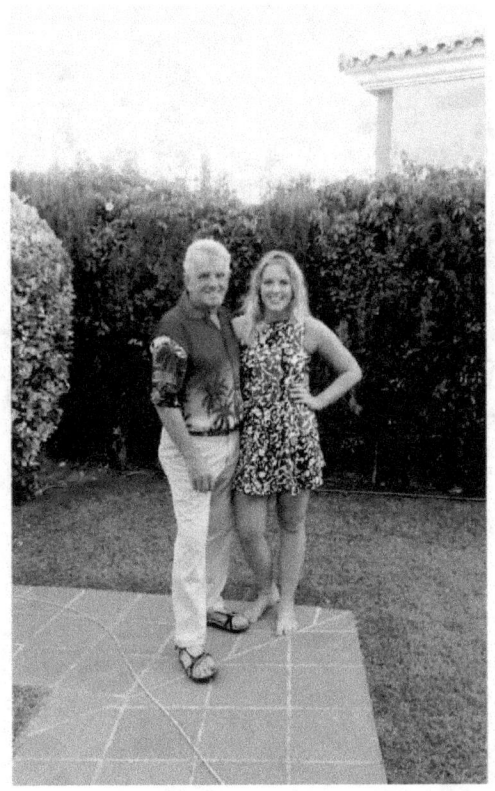

Together; Dad and me in happier times

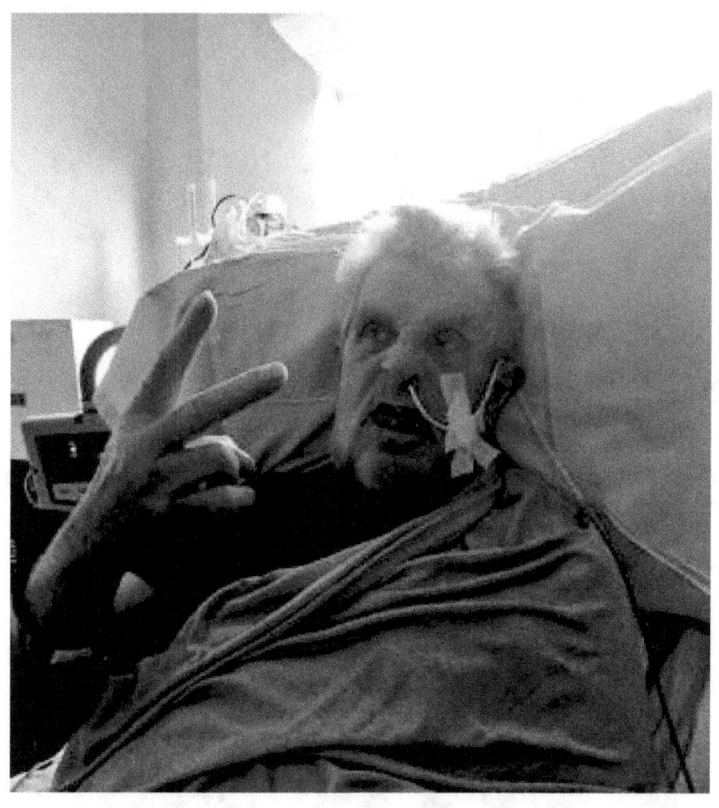

Seen here in defiant mood against cancer two days
after surgery

My father has recently written a short story retelling
his experience of cancer. He asked me to proof read
it, and of course I obliged trying desperately to give
a critical response. However, that was almost
impossible, tears rolling down my face for the first

time; I saw the last 9 months through my Daddy's eyes.

Anyone who knows Martin Read will know that he is a warm, funny and generous man, certain to always be the first to tell an anecdote or to laugh (loudly) at any joke that comes his way. I suppose I want to write this piece almost in response to Dad's story, his aim is to help the patient and mine is to help the loved ones supporting them. If our story can give comfort to just one person faced with this relentless illness, then we have succeeded.

I first knew that Dad was poorly when my Mum casually mentioned a lump in his mouth. In my usual way I pushed it aside and assumed it to be nothing, similar to what my Dad did when he first found it. However, I remember that his first appointment was on a Monday, in which he would get his results. I texted my mum in my afternoon break asking if I should 'prepare myself', to which she replied 'A little bit xxx'.

All the way home I prepared myself to be strong, not to cry and even thought of some cancer based jokes that definitely would have been extremely inappropriate. My parents were in the kitchen, so I sat on the counter as usual and waited for what I knew was coming. My dad had tears in his eyes and blurted out that it was cancer in his tongue and throat. I'm sure that they told me some further details but all I remember is 'don't cry' running through my head. I went to my room, rang my friend Faye and then got ready for bed. I tried to sleep but couldn't and ended up crying on Mums shoulder, feeling as though I was 5 again and needing comfort after a bad dream.

The days went slowly then, for Dad they were filled with doctors' appointments and scans and for me and Mum all we could do was keep positive and only cry when we were with each other. We both decided that to Dad and the world we would be warriors, but with each other we were allowed to show weakness. It was my 19th birthday a few weeks later, I honestly didn't want to celebrate, and I felt that I didn't matter, that it should really all be about him. Faye had written my annual birthday card which of course had us all in floods of tears at the dinner table. I just had to be thankful that he was well

enough to eat, drink and complain about having to
sit through The Tempest (my choice).

Weeks disappeared and it came to operation day, on
Sunday night I said bye, told him I loved him and of
course cried myself to sleep. They left at 6 o clock
the next morning, whilst I woke at 9 and made my
way to school. There waiting was Tilly, a new and
marvellous friend who shared my burden. Both of
our Daddy's have been ill and in her I found great
solace.

That night I decided that I wanted to see him, warts
and all straight out of the operation. My Aunty Cal
had arrived from Belgium in a gracious gesture to
offer comfort to my Mum and I, I know that she
knows this, but we wouldn't have coped without
her. My Mum and Aunty went into the critical care
unit first, whilst I waited anxiously in the waiting
room, where there is actually a lovely 3D picture of
some fields (they almost managed to distract me).
Anyway, my Aunty came out, so it was my turn and
the head nurse took me in her arms and walked me
into the room. I'll never forget how he looked, just

lying there covered in blood, stitches and swelling, I could do nothing but cry.

I next saw him a few days later, sat up and conscious (which was a bloody relief). Still my Dad, but just with a new tongue made from his arm. The poor thing was unable to talk so would write things like 'I'm fed up' on his note pad. This was heart breaking; his low moments were when we had to be strongest. I would joke about his nightie and his socks, to uplift him but mainly to keep myself from crying. To this day I'm glad to say I never cried in front of him (except for recently when he made me read his story).

Another obstacle was how to tell people, my parents told family and the hardest part was the first time they saw dad after they had been told. A prolonged hand shake or hug that you knew meant more than just hello, and a constant tear in everybody's eye. It was easier with family, Aunty Jo and I would hug rather than speak about Dad which for us both was a great comfort. I failed to give my friends the opportunity to support me because I stuck to a 'need to know' basis. However, when I did let them know they were beautifully understanding, concerned and supportive.

Despite my Dad being in hospital, the exhaustion of driving from school after a full day of acting lessons, the heart break of a relationship ending and the longing for my best friend, I refused to stop and wallow in what was happening and just coped. Mum's strength encouraged me and I knew that if she could do it, I could too. The example that my Mother and two gorgeous Aunties showed me increased my strength and enabled me to cope.

I would also like to thank all of the friends in our lives that offered comfort and friendship to me but most importantly to my Mum. The girls took her for drinks and the lads visited Dad as soon as he was home. I never thought that food left on the door step would make me cry but Trish and Sue's parcels always managed to do so.

I am so happy to say that I can now see my Dad again. Through the weight loss, muffled speech and swelling I can see the man that I admire and love. Although he doesn't think it, he is getting stronger every day. As anyone knows who has experienced cancer themselves, it is a slow recovery but thank god it's a recovery! There are many thousands of people that don't get the opportunity to recover, so every time I hear my dad cough, or complain about the pain I thank my lucky stars.

A positive mental attitude, support from loved ones and a lot of hope, can make this 'shitty shit bastard' a lot easier to cope with. I know that it's important to my Dad that the hospital staff are acknowledged. To a complete stranger, nurses and doctors can offer great comfort and I am eternally grateful for the work that they do. I hope that Dad's book will be available for purchase in the near future; all profits will go toward cancer research.

Onwards and upwards, all you can do is put your positive pants on. x